AROMATHERAPY

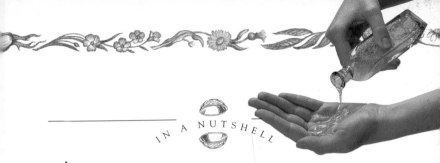

IN A NUTSHELL

AROMATHERAPY
A STEP-BY-STEP
GUIDE

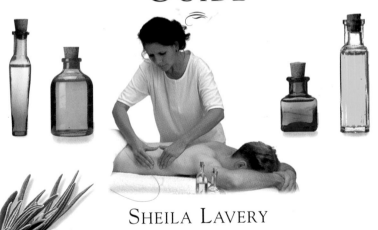

SHEILA LAVERY

ELEMENT

SHAFTESBURY, DORSET • BOSTON, MASSACHUSETTS • MELBOURNE, VICTORIA

First published in
Great Britain in 1997 by
ELEMENT BOOKS LIMITED
Shaftesbury, Dorset, SP7 8BP

Published in the USA in 1997 by
ELEMENT BOOKS INC
160 North Washington Street,
Boston, MA 02114

Published in Australia in 1997 by
ELEMENT BOOKS LIMITED
and distributed by Penguin Australia Ltd
487 Maroondah Highway, Ringwood,
Victoria 3134

Reprinted February, September 1998

NOTE FROM THE PUBLISHER
Any information given in this book is
not intended to be taken as a replacement
for medical advice. Any person with
a condition requiring medical attention
should consult a qualified practitioner
or therapist.

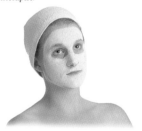

Designed and created with
The Bridgewater Book Company Ltd
ELEMENT BOOKS LIMITED
Managing Editor Miranda Spicer
Senior Commissioning Editor Caro Ness
Production Manager Susan Sutterby
Production Controller Fiona Harrison
Project Editor Katie Worrall

THE BRIDGEWATER BOOK COMPANY LTD
Art Director Peter Bridgewater
Designers Andrew Milne, Jane Lanaway
Page layout Chris Lanaway, Sue Rose
Managing Editor Anne Townley
Picture Research Lynda Marshall
Three dimensional models Mark Jamieson
Photography Ian Parsons, Guy Ryecart
Illustrations Andrew Milne, Andrew Kulman
Text consultants BOOK CREATION SERVICES LTD
Series Editor Karen Sullivan

Printed and bound in Italy by Graphicom S.r.l

British Library Cataloguing in
Publication data available

Library of Congress Cataloging
in Publication data available

ISBN 1–86204–012–5

The publishers wish to thank the
following for the use of pictures: A–Z Botanical
Collection Ltd: pp.22TR, 34TL, 36TL, 38TR,
42TL, 44TL, 50TL; Bridgeman Art Library:
pp.8TL, 8/9; e.t.archive: p.9T; Harry Smith
Collection: pp.30TL, 32TR, 40TL, 46TL,
48TL; Image Bank: pp.11BR, 52B

Special thanks go to:
Tom Aitken, Cheryl Butler, Carly Evans, Julia
Holden, Simon Holden, Stephen Sparshatt
for help with photography

Ken Gross. The Plinth Company Ltd,
Stowmarket, Suffolk
for help with properties

Contents

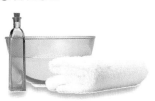

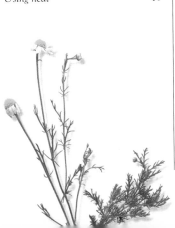

What is aromatherapy?

THE TERM AROMATHERAPY *is used to describe a particular branch of herbal medicine. It is coined from two words, "aroma" meaning pleasant scent and "therapy" meaning a treatment that aims to cure a physical or mental condition. Literally it means treatment using scents. The scents involved are not perfumes but the pure essential oils of plants valued for their therapeutic properties. Treatment involves applying these oils to the body to improve physical, mental, and emotional health.*

ABOVE **Flowers, leaves, herbs, bark, and roots are the five main sources of essential oils.**

LAVENDER

Essential oils are the basic tools of aromatherapy. The oils, which are extracted from plants (*see page 20*), can be used to treat all systems of the body, disturbances of the mind, and imbalances of the emotions. There are many ways to use essential oils. Professional aromatherapists tend to favor massage as the most effective way of getting oils into

ABOVE **For massage essential oils are diluted in vegetable oil.**

the body. Massage also increases the healing potential of aromatherapy. The medicinal properties of the oils and the nurturing power of touch combine to form a potent healing treatment. Massage can be relaxing or energizing, it can

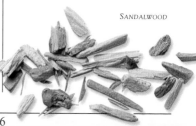

SANDALWOOD

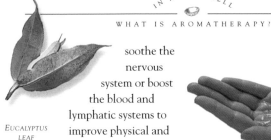

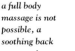

EUCALYPTUS LEAF

soothe the nervous system or boost the blood and lymphatic systems to improve physical and mental functioning.

Not least among its benefits is the way it can ease pain and tension from tense or overworked muscles and lift the spirits. Whenever possible, try to include massage in your home aromatherapy treatments; where this is not possible, use any of the other methods mentioned below and described in greater detail on pages 16–19.

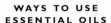

ABOVE *Always warm massage oil in your hands before applying to the skin.*

RIGHT *Where a full body massage is not possible, a soothing back massage is often the next best choice of treatment.*

WAYS TO USE ESSENTIAL OILS

Massage using diluted essential oils.

Steam inhalations using essential oil and hot water.

Vaporizers use heat to release the scent and properties of the oils into the air.

Baths scented with the oils.

Compresses using pieces of cotton soaked in water and essential oils.

Creams, lotions shampoos and shower gels that have essential oils added to them.

Gargles and mouthwashes

Neat Some essential oils can be applied undiluted to the skin.

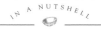

A short history

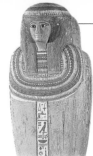

ABOVE *Ancient Egyptians used fragrant oils such as cedarwood, frankincense, and myrrh in the embalming process.*

MOST ANCIENT CULTURES *valued the therapeutic benefits of aromatic plant oils. The ancient Vedic literature of India and historic Chinese medical texts document the importance of scented oils in promoting health and spirituality. Hippocrates, regarded as the "father of medicine," used fragrant fumigations to rid Athens of plague, and Roman soldiers were strengthened by scented oil baths and regular massage. But the richest aromatic traditions belong to the ancient Egyptians. Physicians from all over the world are reputed to have traveled to Egypt to learn aromatic medicine from these masters.*

WESTERN DEVELOPMENTS

Aromatherapy is believed to have come to the Western world at the time of the Crusades. There are records of essential oils being used during the plague in the fourteenth century. But it was during the sixteenth and seventeenth centuries that aromatherapy was most popular. The great European herbalists, including the Englishman, Nicholas Culpeper, wrote avidly about its benefits. During the last two centuries scientists developed a greater understanding of plant oil chemistry.

LAVENDER

BELOW *Four-thousand-year-old papyrus manuscripts record how the Egyptians used aromatic oils for religious and medicinal purposes.*

MODERN PIONEERS

Ironically, scientific research led to the growth of the drug industry and the demise of plant medicine. Then, in the 1920s, a French chemist, René Maurice Gattefossé, became intrigued by the healing potential of essential oils. He discovered that lavender oil quickly healed a burn on his hand and that many essential oils were better antiseptics than their synthetic counterparts. It was Gattefossé who coined the term *aromathérapie*.

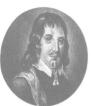

ABOVE **Culpeper listed the properties of many herbs.**

Dr. Jean Valnet

A French army surgeon Dr. Jean Valnet furthered research by using essential oils to treat soldiers wounded in battle. Later he used the oils with great success on patients in a psychiatric hospital. In 1964 Valnet published *Aromathérapie*, which is widely regarded as the bible of aromatherapy.

Marguerite Maury

In the 1950s Madame Marguerite Maury, a beauty therapist, introduced aromatherapy clinics to Britain. She taught beauty therapists how to use essential oils in massage to provide a treatment which was suited to each individual client.

In recent years aromatherapy has developed far beyond beauty therapy. It is now a recognized and important part of complementary healthcare.

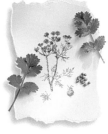

BELOW **Coriander has been used therapeutically for at least 4,000 years.**

How does aromatherapy work?

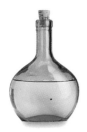

ESSENTIAL OILS *enter the body by inhalation and by absorption through the pores of the skin. They affect the system in three ways: pharmacologically, physiologically, and psychologically, as annotated below.*

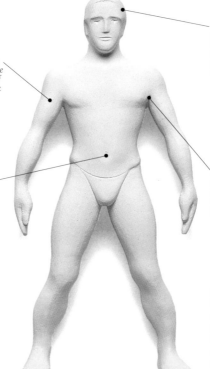

Once inhaled, aromatic signals are sent to the limbic system of the brain where they exert a direct effect on the mind and emotions

The chemical constituents of the oils are carried in the bloodstream to all areas of the body, where they react with body chemistry in a way similar to drugs

Certain oils also have an affinity with particular areas of the body and their properties have a balancing, sedating, or stimulating effect on body systems

After several hours the oils leave the body. Most are exhaled, others are eliminated in urine, feces, and perspiration

LEFT **It can take between 20 minutes and several hours for oils to be absorbed into the body, but on average it takes about 90 minutes.**

HOW DOES IT FEEL?

Depending on the choice of oils and method of treatment, aromatherapy produces any number of sensations. For most people safe treatment is pleasant, enjoyable, and relaxing.

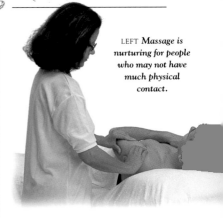

LEFT **Massage is nurturing for people who may not have much physical contact.**

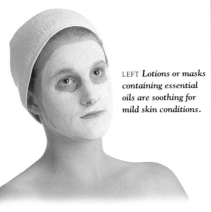

LEFT **Lotions or masks containing essential oils are soothing for mild skin conditions.**

WHO BENEFITS?

People of all ages and levels of health can benefit. It is nurturing for babies and children and it gives many elderly people a feeling of being cared for. Pregnant women and even seriously ill patients can benefit from professional treatment.

WHAT DOES IT TREAT?

Aromatherapy benefits the person rather than their illness. But it has been shown to be particularly good for stress-related problems, muscular and rheumatic pains, digestive disorders, menstrual and menopausal complaints, anxiety, insomnia, and depression.

BELOW **A therapeutic bath is the easiest way to treat yourself at home.**

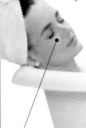

Oils are inhaled and absorbed

Treatment

THIS BOOK *is intended as an introductory guide and as a handbook for self-treatment. Aromatherapy is one of the most enjoyable of all complementary therapies and it is safe and easy to use at home providing you follow certain basic guidelines.*

LEFT *Diluted oils can be applied locally at the site of infection.*

WHEN TO SEE A PROFESSIONAL

Always seek professional treatment for chronic or serious health problems or if a problem becomes severe or persistent. There are certain conditions for which self-treatment is ill-advised.

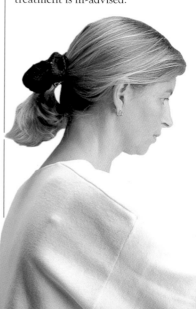

TREATING YOURSELF

Self-treatment is suitable for minor or short-term problems only. For example:

- Minor cuts, burns, and bruises
- Colds, flu, and chest infections
- Mild eczema, dermatitis, rashes, or stings
- Occasional bouts of constipation and diarrhea, hemorrhoids, and indigestion

- Occasional cystitis, painful or irregular periods, and mild PMS
- Short-term anxiety, tension, mild depression, and insomnia
- The conditions listed on pages 53–8

How many sessions are necessary?

The number of treatments required depends on the nature of the problem, the length of time you have had it, and how fast you heal. For relaxation, have as many treatments as you like.

Can I combine treatment with other therapies?

Aromatherapy is compatible with conventional medicine and most other forms of holistic treatment. However, if you are taking medication, it would be wise to consult your doctor and your aromatherapist. Some essential oils are not compatible with homeopathic treatment.

WARNING

Consult a qualified practitioner for advice and treatment:

- If you are pregnant
- Have an allergy
- Have a chronic medical condition such as high blood pressure or epilepsy
- Are receiving medical or psychiatric treatment
- Are taking homeopathic remedies
- When treating babies or very young children

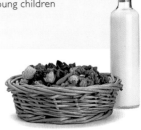

How to find a good quality oil

Choose only those bottles that are labeled "pure essential oil," which are undiluted and unadulterated. If in doubt contact one of the major aromatherapy bodies for a list of approved oil retailers.

ABOVE *Essential oils add a fresh, natural fragrance to lotions and potpourri.*

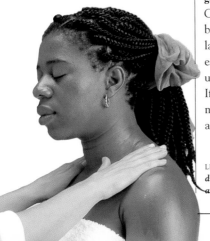

LEFT *If you want to use aromatherapy during pregnancy, it is wise to consult a practitioner.*

BLENDING OILS

Essential oils can be used alone or blended together. Oils are blended for two reasons: to enhance or change their medicinal actions and to create a more sophisticated fragrance. In perfumery many oils are blended together. For therapeutic purposes it is unusual to mix more than four oils together. When blending oils at home it is best to mix no more than two or three oils. This is because blending has been shown to alter the molecular structure of essential oils and you may end up with a blend that acts differently from what you had intended. Make sure the properties of the oils are complementary.

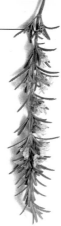

ROSEMARY

YLANG YLANG

BLENDING OILS FOR MASSAGE

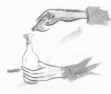

1 Choose a light vegetable base oil such as grapeseed, sweet almond, or sunflower oil.

2 Add your chosen oils a little at a time, shake the bottle, and rub a little into the back of your hand to test. Adjust the quantities until you achieve the blend you want.

3 Mix in about five percent wheat germ oil to preserve the blend.

BLENDING GUIDELINES

Choose two or three oils which you believe complement each other. In general, oils from the same groups (citrus, floral, spicy, etc.) and those which share similar constituents blend well. Using the proportions detailed in the Techniques section, mix a blend using a little of the strongest scented oils and more of the lighter fragrances.

Throughout this book there are recipes for suggested blends. But be guided by your own likes and dislikes. The best blend is usually the one you find most appealing.

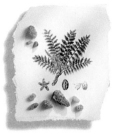

ABOVE *Oils may be extracted from different parts of each plant and blended with other oils to make an individual perfume or remedy.*

BELOW *Once blended, oils may be added to different bases, such as bubble bath, or stored in dark colored bottles.*

CAUTIONS
People with sensitive skin should introduce the oil with caution. NB: Myrrh should not be used during pregnancy. Do not swallow mouthwashes or gargles.

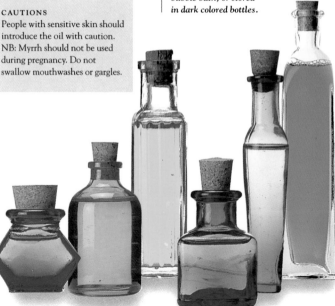

Aromatherapy techniques

THERE ARE MANY *ways to use essential oils at home. Massage and bathing tend to be the most popular and techniques which involve applying oils to the body are usually more effective than inhalation. However there are several other techniques which are particularly beneficial for certain conditions.*

ABOVE **Assemble everything you need for your treatment before you begin.**

BELOW **Use both hands to "mold" the body.**

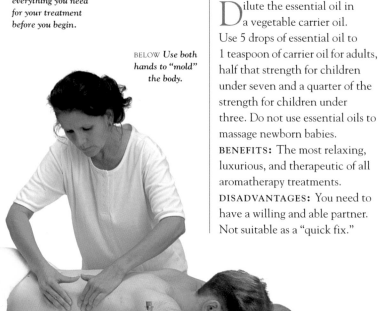

MASSAGE

Dilute the essential oil in a vegetable carrier oil. Use 5 drops of essential oil to 1 teaspoon of carrier oil for adults, half that strength for children under seven and a quarter of the strength for children under three. Do not use essential oils to massage newborn babies.

BENEFITS: The most relaxing, luxurious, and therapeutic of all aromatherapy treatments.

DISADVANTAGES: You need to have a willing and able partner. Not suitable as a "quick fix."

BASIC MASSAGE TECHNIQUES

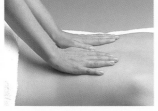

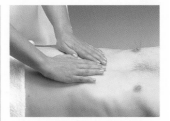

1 **EFFLEURAGE** *Place your hands flat on the bottom of your partner's back. Slide them upward, leaning into the palms to add pressure. At the shoulders, fan your hands out to each side and stroke lightly down each side. Repeat, varying the length of each stroke.*

2 **CIRCLING** *Place both hands on your partner, a few inches apart, and stroke in a wide circular movement. Press into the upward stroke and glide back down. Your arms will cross as you make the circle, so just lift one hand over the other to continue.*

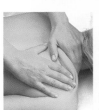

3 **KNEADING** *Place both hands on the area to be massaged with your fingers pointing away from you. Press into the body with the palm of one hand, pick up the flesh between your thumb and fingers, and press it toward the resting hand. Release and repeat with the other hand.*

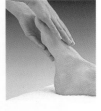

4 *Finish with gentle soothing strokes and end the massage by holding your partner's feet for a few seconds. Holding the feet helps to "ground" the person being massaged and brings them back to reality.*

STEAM INHALATIONS

• Add 3–4 drops of oil to a bowl of boiling water. Bend over the bowl, cover your head with a towel, and breathe deeply for a few minutes. You can also use this method as a facial sauna.

• **Benefits**: Quick and easy, heat increases the benefits of anti-infective oils.

• **Disadvantages**: Not always suitable for asthmatics; dangerous for children.

VAPORIZERS

• Can be electric or a ceramic ring that is heated by a light bulb, but most are ceramic pots warmed by a small candle. Add water and 6–8 drops of oil to the vaporizer. Alternatively, add the oil to a bowl of water and place by a radiator.

• **Benefits**: Scents and purifies the air, clears germs. Good for emotional and breathing problems.

• **Disadvantages**: One of the least effective ways to get oils into the body.

BATHING WITH OILS

For adults add 5–10 drops of essential oil to a full bath. Use less than 4 drops for children over two, and 1 drop for babies. Stir through the water with your hand. For footbaths use 2–3 drops of oil.

BENEFITS: Easy to use; relaxing.
DISADVANTAGES: None.

CREAMS, LOTIONS, AND SHAMPOOS

Add 1–2 drops of essential oil to creams, lotions, and shampoos and massage into the skin or scalp. Choose unscented products made from good quality natural ingredients.

BENEFITS: Convenient for everyday use.
DISADVANTAGES: May irritate sensitive skins.

ABOVE *Adding the oil to running water releases the fragrance.*
RIGHT *Steam inhalations work best for congestion, catarrh, and headaches.*

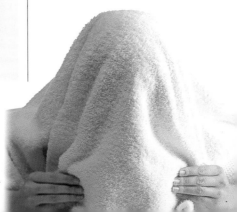

GARGLES AND MOUTHWASHES

Dilute 4–5 drops of essential oil in a teaspoon of brandy. Mix into a glass of warm water and swish around the mouth or use as a gargle. Do not swallow.

BENEFITS: Ideal for throat infections and mouth ulcers.

DISADVANTAGES: Not suitable for children; unpleasant taste.

WARNING

Never take essential oils by mouth. If swallowed accidentally, eat bread, drink plenty of milk, and seek professional help.

Use a clean cotton cloth

Hold in place until pain eases

RIGHT **Hot and cold compresses can be used for pain relief.**

USING NEAT

A few essential oils such as lavender, tea tree, and sandalwood can be applied undiluted to the skin. Most oils should not be used neat as they can cause irritation.

HOT AND COLD COMPRESSES

Add 4–5 drops of essential oil to a bowl of hot or cold water. Soak a folded clean cotton cloth in the water, wring it out, and apply over the affected area. If using a hot compress, cover with a warm towel and repeat when it cools.

• Hot compresses are good for muscle pain, arthritis, rheumatism, toothache, earache, boils, and abscesses.

• Cold compresses are good for headaches, sprains, and swelling.

Essential oils

ESSENTIAL OILS *are extracted from the leaves, flowers, fruit, wood, bark, and roots of plants and trees. They are natural multifaceted chemical compounds, more complex and safer than pharmaceutical drugs, but slower acting so they are best used as a preventive or as a complementary form of treatment.*

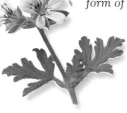

ABOVE **The oils are distilled soon after harvesting as plant material deteriorates rapidly.**

About 150 essential oils have been extracted for use in aromatherapy. Over the next few pages you will find detailed information about 15 of the most useful oils, all of which you can buy from specialist suppliers, healthfood stores, and some large pharmacies.

Each essential oil has a unique fragrance and at least 100 chemical components, which work together to heal mind and body. All the oils are antiseptic, and may have numerous other actions such as being anti-inflammatory, pain-relieving, or antidepressant. Every oil also has a dominant characteristic and is classified accordingly as stimulating, relaxing, or refreshing, for example. A few oils such as lavender are adaptogenic, meaning they do what the body requires of them at the time. Nobody really understands how essential oils affect body functioning in this way.

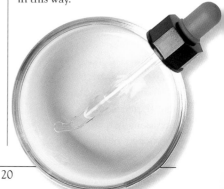

BELOW **Essential oils dissolve in oil or pure alcohol, but not in water.**

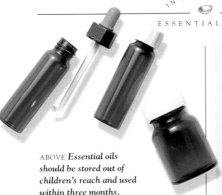

ABOVE *Essential oils should be stored out of children's reach and used within three months.*

HOW THE OILS ARE EXTRACTED

Most pure essential oils are extracted by a process of steam distillation, but other methods such as solvent extraction, enfleurage, and expression are also used. For optimum benefits, essential oils must be extracted from natural raw ingredients and remain as pure as possible.

YOUR 15 OILS

The oils on the following pages have been chosen for their safety, availability, price, and versatility. The blends are made from 10 drops of essential oil; adjust the quantities to suit your choice of technique. Occasionally, additional oils are mentioned in the remedies.

KEY TO DIFFERENT TECHNIQUES

The following symbols are used on pages 23–51.

Massage

Footbath

Bath

Inhalation

Shower

Compress

Vaporizer

Gargle

Neat

Shampoo

Cream or lotion

Mouthwash

Damp cotton wool or dressing

Lavender

LAVANDULA ANGUSTIFOLIA

OF THE SEVERAL *varieties of lavender used medicinally, Lavandula angustifolia is the most important. It is the most versatile, best loved, and most widely therapeutic of all essential oils. Both flowers and leaves are highly aromatic but only the flowers are used to make essential oil.*

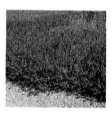

ABOVE **Lavender is a unique oil because it is so versatile; and it blends well with other oils.**

BELOW **The fragrant purple flowers are used to produce pale yellow oil.**

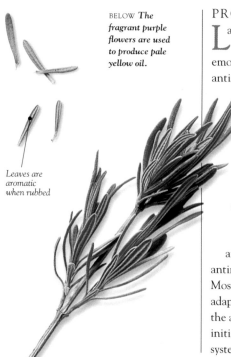

Leaves are aromatic when rubbed

PROPERTIES

Lavender is calming, soothing, antidepressant, and emotionally balancing. Its antiseptic, antibacterial, and painkilling properties make it valuable in treating cuts, wounds, and burns. Because it is also a decongestant, it is effective against colds, flu, and catarrhal conditions. Lavender lowers blood pressure, prevents and eases spasms, is antirheumatic, and also a tonic. Most importantly, lavender is an adaptogen, meaning that it has the ability to restore balance and initiate healing in any body system that is out of balance.

METHODS OF USE

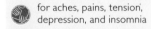 for aches, pains, tension, depression, and insomnia

for digestive problems

for all external uses

for catarrh, colds, flu, and breathing difficulties

for burns, cuts, rashes, and headaches

for sore throats, gums, and bad breath

Blends well with
• Florals such as rose, geranium, ylang ylang, chamomile, and jasmine
• Citrus oils such as orange, lemon, bergamot, and grapefruit
• Rosemary, marjoram, patchouli, clary sage, chamomile, cedarwood, clove, and tea tree

Suggested blends

FOR BACKACHE
4 drops lavender
3 drops eucalyptus
3 drops ginger

FOR EARACHE
2 drops lavender
2 drops tea tree
6 drops chamomile

FOR IRRITABILITY
3 drops lavender
4 drops chamomile
3 drops neroli

MAIN USES

Skin problems such as burns, bruises, spots, allergies, and insect bites benefit. Problems of the nervous system such as tension, depression, insomnia, headaches, stress, and hypertension respond particularly well. It can be used to relieve stomach cramps, nausea, colic, flatulence, and indigestion. It also helps to ease cystitis, relieve asthma, catarrhal conditions, throat infections, and helps to clear bad breath.

ABOVE *Lavender oil increases the therapeutic benefits of any oil with which it is blended.*

CAUTIONS
Usually safe for all age groups, but some hay fever or asthma sufferers may be allergic.

LAVENDER WATER
Pour 1/3 cup rosewater into a bottle and add 30 drops of lavender oil. Shake well, leave in the dark for two weeks. Use as a skin tonic.

Tea tree

MELALEUCA ALTERNIFOLIA

THIS SMALL TREE *or shrub is a traditional remedy among the aboriginal people of Australia. More recently, scientific studies have shown that tea tree oil can combat all types of infection – bacterial, fungal, and viral. It also supports the immune system in its fight against infection.*

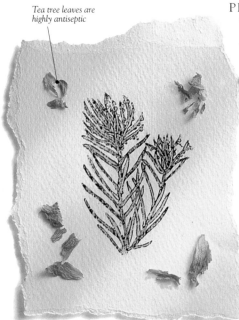

Tea tree leaves are highly antiseptic

PROPERTIES

Primarily an anti-infection oil, tea tree has antifungal, antibacterial, and antiviral properties. It also helps to stop the spread of infection. It is an expectorant that also alleviates inflammation and stimulates the immune system. It helps to heal wounds when applied externally by encouraging the formation of scar tissue and can be used to treat dandruff. Tea tree kills parasites such as fleas and lice and also has cleansing and deodorizing properties.

ABOVE **The leaves and twigs of the shrub are used to produce the oil.**

RIGHT **Tea tree is very good for skin problems and can often be applied neat.**

METHODS OF USE

 for cuts, stings, cold sores, warts, and mouth ulcers

 for throat and mouth infections

 for colds, flu, and respiratory infections

 for vaginal and urinary tract infections

 for athlete's foot, blisters

 for chicken pox and shingles, blisters, rashes

 for sickrooms, colds, breathing problems

 for dandruff

Blends well with
• Lavender, geranium, chamomile, myrrh
• Lemon, rosemary, marjoram, clary sage, pine
• Spice oils such as nutmeg, clove, and cinnamon

Suggested blends
FOR RESPIRATORY INFECTIONS
5 drops tea tree
3 drops pine
2 drops thyme

FOR SPOTS AND ACNE
3 drops bergamot
3 drops lavender
4 drops tea tree

FOR THE MOUTH AND GUMS
5 drops tea tree
5 drops myrrh

MAIN USES

Tea tree is frequently used for skincare problems such as spots and acne, warts, oily skin, athlete's foot, rashes, insect bites, and even burns and blisters. It helps to heal cuts and infected wounds and is effective against dandruff, cold sores, and urinary or genital infections such as cystitis and thrush. It is also valuable in fighting colds, flu, respiratory infections, catarrhal problems, and infectious illnesses. It is also used to stimulate sweating to bring down a fever.

Tea tree is a common ingredient in toothpastes, shampoos, gargles, and deodorants, and in some medicated skincare soaps.

CAUTION
People with sensitive skin should introduce the oil with caution.

RIGHT *A footbath using tea tree oil is ideal for athlete's foot and for soothing aching, blistered feet.*

Rosemary

ROSMARINUS OFFICINALIS

ROSEMARY WAS ONE *of the first herbs to be used medicinally. Traditionally, it was used to ward off evil, offer protection from the plague, and to preserve and flavor meat. It remains a popular culinary and medicinal herb and the oil is regarded as one of the most valuable of all essential oils.*

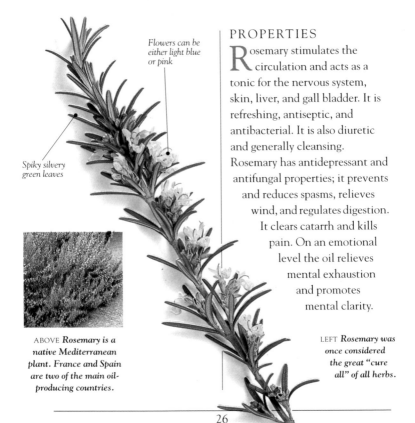

Flowers can be either light blue or pink

Spiky silvery green leaves

PROPERTIES

Rosemary stimulates the circulation and acts as a tonic for the nervous system, skin, liver, and gall bladder. It is refreshing, antiseptic, and antibacterial. It is also diuretic and generally cleansing. Rosemary has antidepressant and antifungal properties; it prevents and reduces spasms, relieves wind, and regulates digestion. It clears catarrh and kills pain. On an emotional level the oil relieves mental exhaustion and promotes mental clarity.

ABOVE **Rosemary is a native Mediterranean plant. France and Spain are two of the main oil-producing countries.**

LEFT **Rosemary was once considered the great "cure all" of all herbs.**

METHODS OF USE

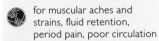 for muscular aches and strains, fluid retention, period pain, poor circulation

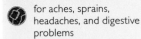 for colds, coughs, headaches, and catarrh

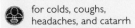 for aches, sprains, headaches, and digestive problems

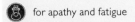 as a tonic, for period pain and fluid retention

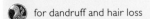 for dandruff and hair loss

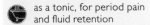 for apathy and fatigue

Blends well with
• Frankincense, petitgrain, basil, thyme, bergamot
• Lavender, peppermint, pine, cedarwood, cypress
• Spice oils such as cinnamon, clove, ginger, black pepper

Suggested blends
FOR CONSTIPATION
4 drops rosemary
4 drops orange
2 drops black pepper

FOR MUSCLE STRAIN
3 drops rosemary
3 drops ginger
4 drops lavender

FOR FLUID RETENTION
4 drops lemon
3 drops rosemary
3 drops patchouli

MAIN USES

An excellent oil for muscle and mental fatigue, coughs and colds, poor circulation, aches, pains, and strains. It is also used for acne, eczema, dandruff, lice, and hair loss. Useful for fluid retention, painful periods, flatulence, indigestion, and constipation. Headaches, low blood pressure, and stress-related disorders also benefit.

ABOVE *The colorless or pale yellow oil has a strong herbal fragrance.*

WIDE AWAKE SHOWER GEL

If you are tired and sluggish in the mornings, mix the following oils with a little of unscented shower gel and work to a lather with a sponge.

• 1 drop rosemary
• 2 drops petitgrain
• 1 drop grapefruit

CAUTIONS
Do not use during pregnancy. Rosemary is not suitable for people with epilepsy or high blood pressure.

Clary sage

SALVIA SCLAREA

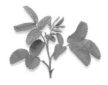

ABOVE *The essential oil is extracted by steam distillation from the flowers and leaves.*

AFFECTIONATELY KNOWN *as "clear eye," clary sage was used in medieval times for clearing foreign bodies from the eyes. Although it is now less well known than common garden sage, clary remains popular in aromatherapy because it is nontoxic and has a pleasant nutty fragrance. The effects of clary sage have been described as "euphoric."*

PROPERTIES

Clary is antidepressant and sometimes described as euphoric. For many people it is simply relaxing and soothing because of its regulating effect on the nervous system. It is also used to help digestion and as a powerful muscle relaxant. Its astringent properties make it beneficial for oily skin and scalp conditions. Clary can also be used to help prevent and arrest convulsions. It is effective against bacteria and may benefit menstruation. As well as lowering blood pressure, clary is also renowned as an aphrodisiac.

Tall flower spikes are supported by yellow and purple bracts

Clary has many of the properties of sage

ABOVE *Clary sage is native to Italy, Syria, and southern France.*

28

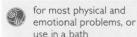

METHODS OF USE

for most physical and emotional problems, or use in a bath

for stress, depression, headaches, and throat infections

for digestive disorders and period pain

for throat infections

for skin conditions

Blends well with
- Lavender, frankincense, sandalwood, cedarwood
- Citrus oils such as lemon, orange, and bergamot
- Geranium, ylang ylang, juniper, coriander

Suggested blends

FOR ANXIETY
4 drops clary sage
3 drops ylang ylang
3 drops lavender

FOR THE MENOPAUSE
5 drops clary sage
2 drops chamomile
3 drops geranium

AS AN APHRODISIAC
4 drops clary sage
4 drops sandalwood
2 drops black pepper

MAIN USES

This oil is most beneficial in treating anxiety, depression, and stress-related problems. It is useful for absent or scanty periods and PMS. It can lower blood pressure and relieve indigestion and flatulence. It helps to ease muscular aches and pains and is good for throat and respiratory infections. Clary sage can also benefit frigidity and impotence.

ABOVE *The oil is colorless with a nutty, herbaceous aroma.*

CAUTIONS

Do not use during pregnancy. Do not use when drinking alcohol as it can make you drunk, drowsy, and can cause nightmares.

RIGHT *Gargling with clary sage is a safe and effective treatment for throat infections.*

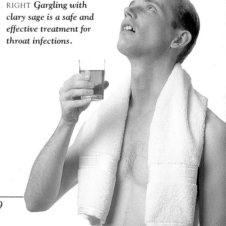

Eucalyptus

EUCALYPTUS GLOBULUS

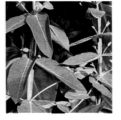

SEVERAL OF THE 700 *species of eucalyptus are used to distil medicinal quality essential oil, but the Australian "blue gum" is by far the most widely used. Eucalyptus is a traditional remedy in Australia and a familiar ingredient in numerous chest rubs and decongestants. In aromatherapy the oil has many varied uses.*

ABOVE **Both old and young leaves are distilled to yield a colorless oil with a distinctive aroma.**

BELOW **Only about 15 of the hundreds of species yield a valuable oil.**

Leaves of mature trees are long, pointed, and yellowy-green

PROPERTIES

Eucalyptus is a powerful antiseptic and renowned decongestant. It also has strong antiviral properties. Eucalyptus alleviates inflammation generally, and is helpful in treating rheumatism. The oil also has insecticidal properties, and can be used to eliminate parasites. It is a diuretic and a deodorant. It stimulates the immune system and is an effective local painkiller, especially for nerve pain. Other properties include its ability to reduce fevers and heal wounds by promoting the formation of scar tissue.

METHODS OF USE

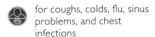 for coughs, colds, flu, sinus problems, and chest infections

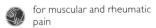 for muscular and rheumatic pain

to purify the air in a sickroom

as a mosquito repellent

for the blisters of chicken pox and shingles, and insect bites

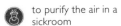 for cuts and wounds

Blends well with
- Peppermint, tea tree
- Rosemary, thyme, lavender
- Cedarwood, lemon, pine

Suggested blends

FOR CHILDHOOD ILLNESSES
3 drops eucalyptus
3 drops chamomile
4 drops lavender

FOR CHEST INFECTIONS
4 drops eucalyptus,
2 drops thyme
2 drops pine
1 drop lavender

WARNING
Do not take internally as ingesting even small amounts can be fatal.

MAIN USES

Used mostly for coughs, colds, chest infections, and sinusitis. It is also valuable in preventing the spread of infection. Eucalyptus soothes muscular aches and pains such as rheumatism and fibrositis. It is also beneficial in treating skin infections, cuts, and blisters, including the blisters associated with genital and oral herpes, chicken pox, and shingles. Urinary tract problems such as cystitis also respond well. When used to treat burns, eucalyptus eases the pain and helps new tissue to form. It helps to prevent and relieve insect bites and is an effective mosquito repellent.

CAUTIONS

Do not take when using homeopathic remedies. Do not use for more than a few days at a time because of risk of toxicity. Do not use on babies or very young children.

RIGHT *Eucalyptus oil is used in ointments, liniments, and cough remedies.*

Geranium

PELARGONIUM GRAVEOLENS

THE FAMILIAR POTTED GERANIUM *has a long history of use in herbal medicine. Over 700 varieties exist and their essential oils differ depending on where the plant is grown. Fresh and floral in fragrance, geranium was traditionally regarded as a feminine oil, a powerful healer and valuable insect repellent.*

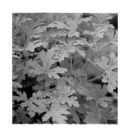

BELOW **Both the fresh leaves and small pink flowers of the plant are distilled for their essential oil.**

The odor of the blossoms superficially resembles that of the rose

The fresh green leaves give the oil its green color

PROPERTIES

Geranium is mentally uplifting and refreshing. It has a balancing effect on the nervous system and is said to be a wonderful antidepressant. The anti-inflammatory, soothing, and astringent properties of geranium account for its success and popularity in skin care. Its antiseptic properties make it useful for cuts and infections. It is also thought to be deodorant, diuretic, and balancing for mind and body. It stimulates the lymphatic system, stops bleeding, and can be used as a tonic for the liver and kidneys.

METHODS OF USE

 for all emotional, circulation, hormonal, and arthritic problems

 for all problems except throat and mouth infections

 for skin complaints

 for sore throat, tonsillitis, and mouth infections

 to deodorize a room

Blends well with
- Lavender, bergamot, rose, rosewood
- Sandalwood, patchouli, frankincense, lemon, jasmine
- Juniper, tea tree, benzoin, basil, black pepper

Suggested blends

FOR HEALTHY SKIN
4 drops geranium
2 drops bergamot
3 drops rose

FOR DEPRESSION
5 drops geranium
3 drops benzoin
2 drops bergamot

FOR PMS
5 drops geranium
3 drops clary sage
2 drops rose

MAIN USES

An effective treatment for numerous skin problems such as acne, diaper rash, burns, blisters, eczema, cuts, and congested pores. Regarded as a feminine oil, geranium is also used to treat PMS and menopausal problems. Its excellent draining properties help to relieve swollen breasts and fluid retention and it stimulates sluggish lymph and blood circulation.

ABOVE *Geranium oil has a light, rose-like fragrance.*

Arthritis and neuralgia are relieved by geranium, and sore throats and mouth ulcers benefit from its antiseptic properties. Geranium is also believed to be emotionally balancing, helping to alleviate apathy, anxiety, stress, hyperactivity, and also depression.

CAUTIONS
May irritate the skin of some hypersensitive individuals. Do not use during the first three months of pregnancy and not at all if there is a history of miscarriage.

Lemon

CITRUS LIMON

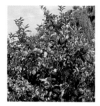

LEMON IS MORE COMMONLY *regarded as a nutritious fruit rather than a healing agent, but it has a history of therapeutic use throughout Europe. The essential oil which is expressed from the fresh peel has many varied applications, making it invaluable in the home aromatherapy kit.*

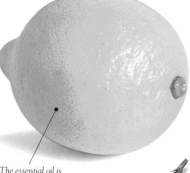

The essential oil is pressed from the outer rind of lemons

Evergreen, oval leaves

ABOVE **The lemon tree is an attractive tree of up to 20ft.(6m) with fragrant flowers, oval leaves, and bright yellow fruit.**

PROPERTIES

The most important property of lemon is its ability to stimulate the body's defenses to fight infection. The oil is also refreshing and has a tonic effect on the circulation. It is antiseptic and a wonderful antibacterial. Lemon is astringent, diuretic, and laxative and has the ability to arrest bleeding. It may also lower blood pressure, prevent and relieve rheumatism, and reduce a fever. Because it counteracts acidity in the body, lemon can also help to maintain a healthy acid/alkaline balance.

METHODS OF USE

 as a tonic and for most health problems

 as a room refresher or mood enhancer

 on affected skin, cuts, gums, or nosebleeds and neat on warts

 for circulation and as a tonic

 for cold and flu-like conditions

 over the site of acid indigestion or arthritic pain

Blends well with
• Lavender, rose, ylang ylang, neroli, chamomile
• Juniper, benzoin, frankincense, black pepper, basil, sandalwood
• Other citrus oils such as orange, lime, bergamot

Suggested blends
FOR CIRCULATION
6 drops lemon
3 drops cypress
4 drops ylang ylang

FOR FATIGUE
4 drops lemon
2 drops black pepper
4 drops sandalwood

FOR DEPRESSION
2 drops lemon
3 drops rose
5 drops sandalwood

MAIN USES

Lemon kills infection and stops bleeding in minor cuts and nosebleeds. It can be used to remove warts, corns, and similar growths and also helps to clear greasy skin, acne, and herpes blisters. It is beneficial in treating inflamed or diseased gums and mouth ulcers and useful for acid indigestion, arthritis, and rheumatism. It is often used to treat varicose veins, poor circulation, and high blood pressure. Lemon helps to clear colds, flu, and bronchitis. It can be used against all types of infection. Lemon dispels depression and indecision. Lemon can be used as a mild skin bleach for freckles and it also makes an effective insect repellent.

ABOVE *The greenish yellow oil has a fresh citrus fragrance.*

CAUTIONS

Can irritate sensitive skin. Do not use before sunbathing. Use only very diluted in massage and bath blends, and not for more than a few days at a time.

Peppermint

MENTHA PIPERITA

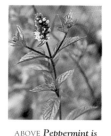

PEPPERMINT *is best known as a remedy for digestive problems. It was used as such by the Romans and possibly the ancient Egyptians. Apart from its many therapeutic applications it is also used as a humane form of pest control. Peppermint grows throughout Europe but most oil comes from the United States.*

ABOVE **Peppermint is a perennial herb that is grown throughout the world.**

Flowering peppermint is distilled to make essential oil

Fresh peppermint leaves

PROPERTIES

Peppermint is refreshing and stimulating. It tones and settles the digestive system, relieves flatulence, and reduces spasms. It also helps to tone the stomach, liver, and intestines, while strengthening and toning the nervous system. It is a valuable expectorant, a painkiller, an antiseptic, and it relieves itching. Peppermint can reduce fevers in two ways: it induces sweating and it has a cooling effect on the body. Peppermint also promotes clarity of thought. It is often used as an emergency treatment for shock, because of its stimulant properties.

METHODS OF USE

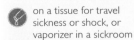 on a tissue for travel sickness or shock, or vaporizer in a sickroom

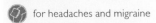 for headaches and migraine

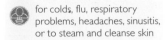 for colds, flu, respiratory problems, headaches, sinusitis, or to steam and cleanse skin

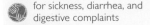 for sickness, diarrhea, and digestive complaints

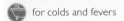 for colds and fevers

 footbath for chilblains

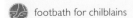 for bad breath

Blends well with
• Lavender, chamomile, rosemary, lemon
• Eucalyptus, benzoin, sandalwood, marjoram
• Other mints such as spearmint

Suggested blends

FOR VOMITING
3 drops lavender
4 drops peppermint
3 drops chamomile

FOR HEADACHES
3 drops peppermint
4 drops lavender
3 drops rose

FOR BAD BREATH
5 drops peppermint
3 drops bergamot
2 drops myrrh

MAIN USES

Most commonly used for indigestion, diarrhea, nausea, vomiting, stomach cramps, and travel sickness. It is also used for bronchitis, colds, flu, acne, and congested skin. Beneficial for toothache, headaches, some migraines, and as an emergency remedy for shock. Muscle and mental fatigue are both relieved by peppermint and it also freshens bad breath.

ABOVE
Peppermint oil has a strong minty fragrance.

CAUTIONS

Do not use during pregnancy. May sensitize or irritate the skin in some people. Do not use while taking homeopathic remedies. Use in moderation.

PEPPERMINT INHALATION

For colds, flu, and respiratory disorders, use the oil alone or blended with other expectorant and antiseptic oils. Try:
• sandalwood and/or pine for chest infections
• eucalyptus/lavender/sandalwood for flu and catarrh

Petitgrain

CITRUS AURANTIUM

PETITGRAIN IS *often regarded as a cheaper alternative to the exquisite essential oil, neroli. Both oils come from the bitter orange tree and share similar properties and fragrances. But where neroli comes from the blossom, fresh and flowery petitgrain is distilled from the leaves and twigs.*

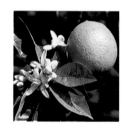

Petitgrain oil used to be extracted from the tiny unripe oranges

PROPERTIES

Petitgrain is a soothing oil that can be refreshing or relaxing depending on which oils it is blended with. It is a valuable antidepressant, which also strengthens and supports the nervous system and acts as a general tonic. It helps to tone the digestive system and is able to control and reduce spasms in the body, especially in the digestive system. Petitgrain is a deodorant and a gentle antiseptic. It also helps to control the overproduction of sebum in the skin and is a refreshing bath oil.

ABOVE **Citrus aurantium** *is native to southern China and northeast India.*

Fresh leaves used in distillation

METHODS OF USE

to refresh, relax, uplift, or for convalescence

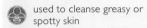
for most emotional and physical conditions

used to cleanse greasy or spotty skin

for depression or anxiety states

for hair care

for skin problems

Blends well with
• Geranium, ylang ylang, chamomile, oakmoss, jasmine
• Bergamot, lemon, orange, neroli
• Clary sage, clove, rosemary, lavender, juniper

Suggested blends

FOR ANXIETY
4 drops petitgrain
3 drops geranium
3 drops sandalwood

FOR INSOMNIA
3 drops petitgrain
4 drops lavender
3 drops ylang ylang

FOR DRY SKIN
2 drops petitgrain
5 drops chamomile
3 drops rose

RIGHT **Petitgrain can be used for the treatment of exhaustion and depression.**

MAIN USES

Ideal for many greasy skin and scalp conditions, especially acne and greasy hair. It is also sometimes used to control excessive perspiration and flatulence. Petitgrain is valuable for many stress-related problems such as nervous exhaustion and insomnia. It is helpful during convalescence or periods of exhaustion and feeling "run down." Feelings of apathy, irritability, mild depression, and anxiety can all be alleviated by refreshing petitgrain. The oil is also believed to have a comforting effect on those who feel sad and lonely.

ABOVE **The pale to deep yellow oil is a refreshing mix of floral and citrus notes.**

CAUTIONS
None known.

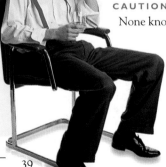

Ylang ylang

CANANGA ODORATA VAR. GENUINA

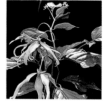

THE NAME OF THIS OIL *means "flower of flowers," which suits its sweet fragrance. It is distilled from the flowers of a small tree that grows in Madagascar. The large fragrant flowers can be mauve, pink, or yellow. The yellow flowers are believed to produce the best oil.*

ABOVE **Oil is extracted from the fresh flowers.**

PROPERTIES

Ylang ylang is used as a sedative and an antidepressant, and is widely regarded as a "euphoric." It is also attributed with aphrodisiac properties. On a physical level it is antiseptic and inhibits the spread of infection. It acts as a tonic for the nervous and circulatory systems, it slows a rapid heart beat and breathing, and can help lower blood pressure. It also controls the production of sebum and may be used to help balance and regulate body functions generally.

ABOVE **The fresh leaves of the tropical ylang ylang tree, which grows up to 65ft(19.8m) high.**

METHODS OF USE

 for most emotional and physical problems

 for relaxation, and most emotional and physical problems

 for skin and hair care

 for shock and other emotional states, inhaled from a tissue

Blends well with
• Lavender, jasmine, sandalwood, chamomile, bergamot, rose, rosewood
• Patchouli, frankincense
• Citrus oils such as lemon and bergamot

Suggested blends
FOR STRESS
4 drops lavender
3 drops ylang ylang
3 drops clary sage
FOR HIGH BLOOD PRESSURE
2 drops ylang ylang
5 drops chamomile
3 drops lavender
FOR OILY SKIN
3 drops ylang ylang
3 drops lemon
4 drops geranium

RIGHT *The lingering sweet fragrance of ylang ylang combined with its reputation as an aphrodisiac makes it a popular ingredient in perfumes.*

MAIN USES

Ylang ylang is good for skin complaints, especially oily or irritated skin and acne, as well as bites and stings. Ylang ylang was an ingredient in the Victorian hair preparation, macassar oil, and can still be used as a scalp tonic to promote hair growth and balance sebum production in both dry and greasy scalps. Good for reducing blood pressure and for slowing breathing and heart rate in cases of shock, panic, or rage. Depression, anxiety, tension, and stress-related insomnia can also be alleviated by ylang ylang. The oil can also be used to treat sexual problems.

ABOVE *Citrus oils help to tone down the intense fragrance of this pale yellow oil.*

CAUTIONS
Can cause nausea or headaches in high concentrations. May irritate some hypersensitive people. Remember to keep all essential oils out of children's reach.

Roman chamomile

CHAMAEMELUM NOBILE

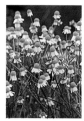

CHAMOMILE IS ONE of the most gentle of all essential oils, which makes it particularly suitable for children. There are many varieties of chamomile, but two of the most commonly used in aromatherapy are Roman chamomile and German chamomile. Both varieties share many properties and uses. Types of chamomile vary from country to country.

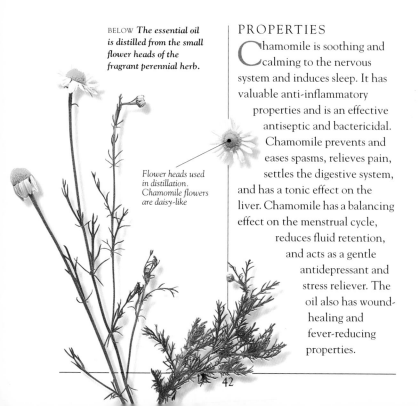

BELOW *The essential oil is distilled from the small flower heads of the fragrant perennial herb.*

Flower heads used in distillation. Chamomile flowers are daisy-like

PROPERTIES

Chamomile is soothing and calming to the nervous system and induces sleep. It has valuable anti-inflammatory properties and is an effective antiseptic and bactericidal. Chamomile prevents and eases spasms, relieves pain, settles the digestive system, and has a tonic effect on the liver. Chamomile has a balancing effect on the menstrual cycle, reduces fluid retention, and acts as a gentle antidepressant and stress reliever. The oil also has wound-healing and fever-reducing properties.

METHODS OF USE

 for tired or fretful babies, toddlers, stressed adults

 for pain, cystitis, boils, abscesses, or infected wounds

 for skin and eye problems

 for muscular pain, menstrual problems, insomnia, and stress

Blends well with
• Lavender, ylang ylang, clary sage
• Bergamot, rose, neroli, geranium
• Patchouli, lemon, basil, sandalwood, rosemary

Suggested blends
FOR BROKEN VEINS
4 drops chamomile
2 drops lemon
4 drops rose

FOR LOSS OF APPETITE
4 drops chamomile
4 drops bergamot
3 drops myrrh

FOR EARACHE
5 drops chamomile
2 drops basil
3 drops rose

MAIN USES

Calms distressed or colicky babies and relieves teething pain and earache. Also an important oil for treating insomnia, anxiety, and stress. Beneficial for digestive upsets such as indigestion, nausea, and flatulence. Many types of dull, aching pain such as headaches, toothache, menstrual pain, muscular aches and pains, arthritis, rheumatism, and neuralgia respond well to chamomile. It is a gentle but effective treatment for cuts and burns and all manner of skin problems, including skin rashes, inflammation, boils, spots, allergies, insect bites, and chilblains. Chamomile is also used to treat eye problems such as eyestrain and conjunctivitis.

CAUTIONS
Do not use in the first three months of pregnancy. Can cause dermatitis in some people. No known risk of toxicity.

LEFT *Chamomile yields a pale blue liquid which turns yellow on keeping.*

Frankincense

BOSWELLIA CARTERI

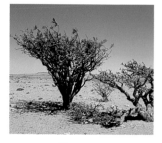

ABOVE **The tree is lavishly colored with small leaves and pale pink or white flowers.**

FRANKINCENSE IS *a wonderfully calming and fragrant oil. Throughout history it has been used for religious and medicinal purposes. It is still regarded as a deeply spiritual oil, but is also beneficial for treating many physical and emotional problems. Frankincense is sometimes known as olibanum.*

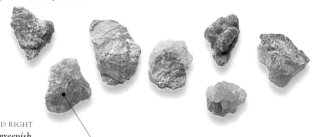

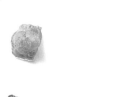

BELOW AND RIGHT **The spicy greenish or pale yellow oil is extracted from the resin of a small tree that grows in north African and some Arab countries.**

Gum resin is a natural product of the tree

PROPERTIES

Slows and deepens the breathing, relaxes mind and body. It is antiseptic, astringent, anti-inflammatory, an immune stimulant, and it encourages wound healing. Frankincense is also an expectorant and a nerve and uterine tonic. It benefits menstruation and digestion.

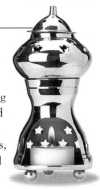

METHODS OF USE

 for cystitis and most urinary problems

 for most physical and emotional problems

 for meditation, anxiety, breathing difficulties

 for colds, flu, and respiratory infections

 for skin problems

 for cuts, scars, and blemishes

Blends well with
• Geranium, lavender, sandalwood, pine, cedarwood, rose, neroli, bergamot
• Spices such as cinnamon and black pepper
• Citrus oils such as orange and lemon

Suggested blends
FOR PANIC ATTACKS
4 drops lavender
4 drops frankincense
2 drops marjoram
FOR MEDITATION
6 drops frankincense
2 drops ylang ylang
2 drops bergamot
FOR AGING SKIN
3 drops frankincense
4 drops rose
3 drops clary sage

RIGHT *Frankincense oil has a fresh, slightly camphorous scent.*

MAIN USES

Frankincense is helpful in treating many respiratory and catarrhal conditions such as asthma, colds, chest infections, and chronic bronchitis. It also has many uses in skin care including the treatment of cuts, scars and blemishes, and inflammation. It is recommended for easing wrinkles and for giving tone to slack or aging skin. As a nerve tonic it benefits anxiety, depression, and nervous tension among other stress-related problems. Cystitis, hemorrhoids, irregular or heavy periods, and nosebleeds also benefit from the healing properties of frankincense.

ABOVE *Using a vaporizer is the ideal way to benefit from frankincense's calming, expectorant, and meditative properties.*

CAUTIONS
Frankincense is safe to use during pregnancy and there are no known risks associated with its external use. As with all essential oils, keep out of children's reach and never take internally.

Rose

ROSA DAMASCENA, ROSA CENTIFOLIA

TWO TYPES OF ROSE, *Damask and Cabbage, are used to produce most of the rose oil used in aromatherapy. They are slightly different in color and fragrance but have similar properties and uses. Rose oil is expensive but you need only use a little to benefit from its many therapeutic properties.*

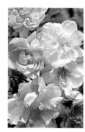

ABOVE **The essential oil is distilled from the fresh rose petals.**

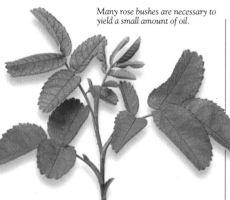

Many rose bushes are necessary to yield a small amount of oil.

ABOVE **The traditionally "feminine" rose produces an oil particularly beneficial for women.**

PROPERTIES

Rose oil has an amazingly complex chemistry and its benefits are many and varied. It is a renowned aphrodisiac, a sedative, and a tonic with notable antidepressant properties. It is an antiseptic, powerful against both viruses and bacteria. Rose oil astringes and tones the blood and acts as a tonic for the heart, liver, stomach, and uterus.

Traditionally regarded as a feminine oil, it has a remarkable affinity with the female reproductive system. It helps to regulate the menstrual cycle and associated emotional problems. Rose also regulates the stomach and especially the appetite. It prevents and relieves spasms in the digestive system and also acts as a laxative. It is toning and soothing to the skin, stops bleeding, and brings about wound healing by encouraging the formation of scar tissue. Additionally, it helps to detoxify the blood and organs.

METHODS OF USE

 for most emotional and physical problems

 for most emotional and physical problems, especially sexual or reproductive system problems

 for emotional problems

 for headaches, conjunctivitis, nausea, and stomach problems

 for all skin conditions

Blends well with
• Most oils, especially clary sage, sandalwood, geranium, bergamot, patchouli, ylang ylang

Suggested blends
FOR HAY FEVER
3 drops rose
2 drops tea tree
5 drops lavender

FOR CHAPPED SKIN
4 drops rose
3 drops chamomile
3 drops sandalwood

FOR GRIEF
4 drops rose
2 drops frankincense
4 drops chamomile

MAIN USES

Soothes and heals cracked, chapped, sensitive, dry, inflamed, or allergy-prone skin. Broken veins, aging or wrinkled skin also benefit. It is used to improve circulation, alleviate constipation and nausea, and treat stomach problems such as peptic ulcer. Rose lifts depression, especially PMS or post-natal depression, and benefits stress-related conditions such as insomnia and nervous tension. It is also useful in treating headaches, earache, and conjunctivitis. It is an important choice for irregular or painful periods and is believed to aid conception. Hay fever, asthma, and coughs are also soothed by the scent of rose.

CAUTIONS
Do not use during the first three months of pregnancy and not at all if there is a history of miscarriage.

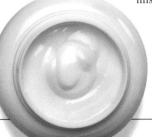

LEFT *Rose has a gentle but powerful regulating effect on the skin which makes it a popular ingredient in numerous commercial skin creams and lotions.*

Patchouli

POGOSTEMON CABLIN

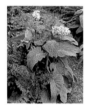

THE DISTINCTIVE *earthy aroma of patchouli is one that you either love or hate. Since smell is so important to the success of aromatherapy, only use the oil if you like its fragrance. For those who do, the oil has many valuable uses and is especially pleasant when used as part of a blend.*

ABOVE **The soft green leaves of the bushy plant are fermented and dried before the essential oil is extracted by steam distillation.**

RIGHT **Patchouli is a member of the same family as basil and sage.**

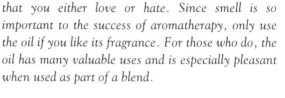

Patchouli leaves are soft and furry

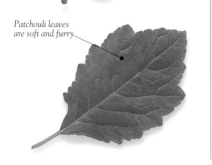

PROPERTIES

Astringent, antiviral, antiseptic and anti-inflammatory. In sickness it brings down fevers, prevents the spread of infection and disease, and reduces the incidence of vomiting. Patchouli soothes and settles the digestive system and acts as a tonic for the nervous system and the body generally. It counteracts the effects of poison and acts as a diuretic. Patchouli has fungicidal and deodorant actions, it is a cell regenerator, and it promotes wound healing. It is also an important antidepressant and is reputed to be an aphrodisiac.

METHODS OF USE

 for cellulite, fluid retention, emotional and stress-related problems

 for most emotional and physical problems

 for emotional and stress-related problems

 for skin care

 dab on affected spots

 for hair care

Blends well with
• Rose, geranium, bergamot, neroli, ylang ylang, lemon
• Sandalwood, clary sage, clove, cedarwood, lavender

Suggested blends

FOR WRINKLES
2 drops patchouli
3 drops lemon
5 drops rose

FOR WOUNDS
3 drops patchouli
4 drops lavender
3 drops tea tree

FOR MOODINESS
2 drops patchouli
3 drops lemon
5 drops geranium

RIGHT *As well as imparting fragrance, the oil is believed to help prevent the spread of disease.*

MAIN USES

Among its many uses patchouli is valued in the treatment of depression, anxiety, nervous exhaustion, lack of interest in sex, and stress-related problems. Minor skin conditions such as chapped or cracked skin and open pores also respond well and it is effective in treating more serious skin problems such as acne, eczema, and dermatitis. Patchouli is one of the few oils recommended for cellulite. It is used with some success in the treatment of fluid retention and is one of the best choices for fungal infections on the skin. Hair and scalp problems such as dandruff and greasy hair can also benefit.

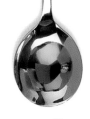

ABOVE *The essential oil is earthy in appearance and fragrance. Dark amber in color with a strong musty-sweet aroma, it is widely used in food and drink production to mask unpleasant tastes and smells.*

CAUTIONS
None known.

Sandalwood

SANTALUM ALBUM

THE SWEET *woody oriental smell of sandalwood is one of the most appealing fragrances of all essential oils, which explains its traditional use as a perfume and incense. The best sandalwood oil comes from India where it has been used for at least 4,000 years for medicinal and religious purposes.*

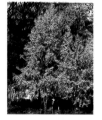

ABOVE **The oil is extracted by steam distillation mainly from the heartwood of mature sandalwood trees which grow in India. Only trees over 30 years old are suitable for essential oil production.**

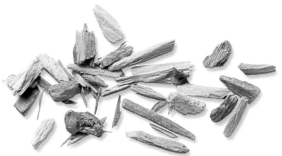

PROPERTIES

Sandalwood is an antiseptic, especially effective for the urinary system. It is also bactericidal and astringent and a trusted insect repellent. It relieves fluid retention, clears catarrh, and encourages wound healing. Although it is a sedative, it also acts as a general tonic for the body. The oil contains constituents that soothe the stomach, reduce spasms, especially in the digestive system, and reduce inflammation. Sandalwood is antidepressant and generally calming to the nervous system. Its aphrodisiac properties are widely acclaimed.

ABOVE **Dry sandalwood chippings impregnated with the sweet woody fragrance can be used as incense.**

METHODS OF USE

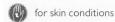 for skin conditions

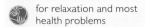 for relaxation and most health problems

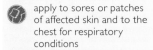 apply to sores or patches of affected skin and to the chest for respiratory conditions

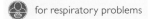 for respiratory problems

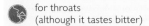 for throats (although it tastes bitter)

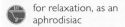 for relaxation, as an aphrodisiac

Blends well with
• Lavender, rose, ylang ylang, geranium, chamomile
• Patchouli, bergamot, frankincense, black pepper, benzoin
• Tea tree, juniper, myrrh, cypress

Suggested blends

FOR HORMONAL BALANCE
3 drops sandalwood
4 drops clary sage
3 drops lavender

FOR SUNBURN
3 drops sandalwood
3 drops lavender
4 drops chamomile

TO STRENGTHEN THE
IMMUNE SYSTEM
4 drops sandalwood
2 drops tea tree
4 drops lavender

MAIN USES

Sandalwood has always been used to treat respiratory conditions and is still effective for bronchitis, dry coughs, and sore throats. It has also proved itself an effective antiseptic for all urinary disorders, especially disorders of the urinary tract such as cystitis. Skin problems such as dry chapped skin, acne, psoriasis, eczema, and shaving rash can also benefit from its soothing, rehydrating, and antiseptic action.

The fragrance can also help to lift depression and banish feelings of anxiety and sexual disinterest.

CAUTIONS
None known.

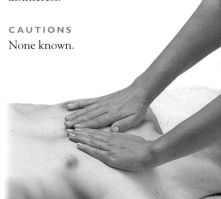

BELOW *As a reputed aphrodisiac, sandalwood is an essential ingredient in a sensual massage blend.*

Home use

ESSENTIAL OILS *make a pleasant alternative to the usual items in the home or travel first aid kit. For such basic care you need invest in only six or seven multi-purpose oils. Keep a ready supply of base oil, cotton wool, cotton cloth, sticking plasters, and bandages. Aromatherapy oils should always be kept out of reach of children, but they can be used successfully for many accidents and childhood ailments.*

ESSENTIAL ITEMS FOR THE HOME

- tea tree
- lavender
- chamomile
- lemon
- eucalyptus
- peppermint
- rosemary
- vegetable oil for blending
- cotton wool/tissues
- mixing bottle
- cotton for compresses
- bandages/plasters
- vaporizer

PLAY SAFE

Do not expect to use essential oils to deal with conditions that would normally require medical attention. In all cases of serious shock, wounds, or injuries call a physician and stay with the patient until he or she arrives.

ABOVE **Applying an aromatherapy oil before doing stretching exercises can help you relax.**

BELOW **This basic first aid kit is ideal for most everyday problems.**

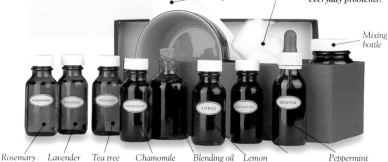

Cotton compress

Cotton wool

Mixing bottle

Rosemary   Lavender   Tea tree   Chamomile   Blending oil   Lemon   Peppermint

Common ailments

HERE ARE *a few of the common health problems that you should be able to treat at home with considerable success. Remember: if symptoms persist or deteriorate, consult a professional aromatherapist or see your physician.*

ALLERGIES
Choose calming oils such as lavender (*pp.22–3*) and chamomile (*pp.42–3*). Also rose (*pp.46–7*), sandalwood (*pp.50–51*), and ylang ylang (*pp.40–41*). Use in massage, baths, compresses, inhalations, and lotions depending on the nature of the allergy.

ANEMIA
Lemon (*pp.34–5*), thyme, and chamomile (*pp.42–3*) in massage oil and in a bath.

ARTHRITIS
Painkilling oils such as chamomile (*pp.42–3*), lavender (*pp.22–3*), and rosemary (*pp.26–7*) in a bath, in local massage, and as a compress on affected area. Black pepper, ginger, and marjoram improve circulation.

ATHLETE'S FOOT
A foot bath with tea tree oil (*pp.24–5*), eucalyptus (*pp.30–31*), patchouli (*pp.48–9*), myrrh, and/or lavender (*pp.22–3*) is effective as all the oils are soothing and antifungal. Also add to unscented skin lotion.

CELLULITE
A blend of geranium (*pp.32–3*) and rosemary (*pp.26–7*) or grapefruit, juniper or cypress used in massage and skin lotion, or add to a bath and use a loofah to stimulate the tissues.

CHILBLAINS

Lemon (*pp.34–5*), lavender (*pp.22–3*), chamomile (*pp.42–3*), cypress, peppermint (*pp.36–7*), or black pepper in massage, in a bath or footbath, or dabbed on the affected area.

COLD SORES

Eucalyptus (*pp.30–31*), bergamot, lemon (*pp.34–5*), or tea tree (*pp.24–5*) are effective. Dab on tea tree (*pp.24–5*) neat or mixed with vodka before the blisters come out. Alternate its use with lavender (*pp.22–3*) to soothe.

COLDS

Lavender (*pp.22–3*), eucalyptus (*pp.30–31*), and tea tree (*pp.24–5*), or rosemary (*pp.26–7*) and peppermint (*pp.36–7*), used in a bath or steam inhalation. A bath using lavender (*pp.22–3*) and marjoram helps reduce aches and feverishness.

COUGHS

Steam inhalation using tea tree (*pp.24–5*), thyme, eucalyptus (*pp.30–31*), lavender (*pp.22–3*), or frankincense (*pp.44–5*). Sandalwood (*pp.50–51*) is good for dry coughs. It also works well massaged into the chest and throat.

CYSTITIS

Chamomile (*pp.42–3*), sandalwood (*pp.50–51*), lavender (*pp.22–3*), frankincense (*pp.44–5*), or tea tree (*pp.24–5*) in baths and washes at least once a day. Use a weak dilution; about 1 percent in boiled and cooled water as a compress.

DANDRUFF

Rosemary (*pp.26–7*), cedarwood, tea tree (*pp.24–5*), or patchouli (*pp.48–9*) massaged into the scalp, added to unscented shampoos, and used in the final rinse when you are washing your hair.

DEPRESSION

For depression with sleeplessness use lavender (*pp.22–3*), sandalwood (*pp.50–51*), chamomile (*pp.42–3*), clary sage (*pp.28–9*), or ylang ylang (*pp.40–41*). With lethargy use bergamot, geranium (*pp.32–3*), rose (*pp.46–7*). With anxiety try ylang ylang (*pp.40–41*) and neroli. Massage

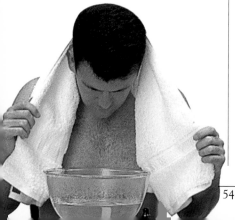

is best, where possible. Otherwise use the oils in the bath or in a vaporizer.

DIARRHEA

Chamomile (*pp.42–3*), lavender (*pp.22–3*), and/or peppermint (*pp.36–7*) added to a bath or massaged over the abdomen. Eucalyptus (*pp.30–31*) is helpful if the diarrhea is caused by a viral infection.

ECZEMA

Lavender (*pp.22–3*), chamomile (*pp.42–3*), sandalwood (*pp.50–51*), rose (*pp.46–7*), melissa, or geranium (*pp.32–3*) in a bath and massage. Add the oils to unscented skin lotion or aqueous cream and rub into the skin. A cool compress can help to soothe irritated patches.

FAINTING

Put a couple of drops of peppermint (*pp.36–7*), lavender (*pp.22–3*), or rosemary (*pp.26–7*) on a tissue to inhale or hold an open bottle containing one of these essential oils under the person's nose.

GINGIVITIS

(Inflammation of the gums) Mouthwashes made with tea tree (*pp.24–5*) or thyme can kill the bacteria that cause infection. Add myrrh for healing and orange to strengthen the gums.

GLANDULAR FEVER

Tea tree oil (*pp.24–5*) is antiviral and strengthens the immune system. Use in a bath and in massage.

HAIR LOSS
AND BALDNESS

Lavender (*pp.22–3*), rosemary (*pp.26–7*), sage, cedarwood, patchouli (*pp.48–9*), or ylang ylang (*pp.40–41*) massaged into the scalp and added to mild unfragranced shampoos.

HANGOVER

Lavender (*pp.22–3*), grapefruit, rosemary (*pp.26–7*), juniper, fennel, or sandalwood (*pp.50–51*) in a bath, in unscented shower gel as an inhalation, or in a vaporizer.

HAY FEVER

Chamomile (*pp.42–3*) in the bath and in massage. Steam or dry inhalations

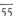

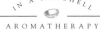

of lavender (*pp.22–3*) and/or eucalyptus (*pp.30–31*) for sneezing and runny nose. Also use in a bath.

HEADACHES 🍃

Neat lavender (*pp.22–3*) rubbed into the temples, forehead, or back of the neck. Add peppermint (*pp.36–7*) if you want to stay alert. Inhalations of lavender (*pp.22–3*), peppermint (*pp.36–7*), or eucalyptus (*pp.30–31*).

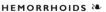

HEMORRHOIDS 🍃

Frankincense (*pp.44–5*), geranium (*pp.32–3*), or juniper used in a bath, in a skin lotion, or on a cool compress. If constipation is part of the problem, massage the abdomen with rosemary (*pp.26–7*).

INDIGESTION 🍃

Gently massage chamomile (*pp.42–3*), lavender (*pp.22–3*), peppermint (*pp.36–7*), rosemary (*pp.26–7*), or clary sage (*pp.28–9*) over the stomach or apply as a hot compress.

INFLUENZA 🍃

Add eucalyptus (*pp.30–31*), lavender (*pp.22–3*), peppermint (*pp.36–7*), or

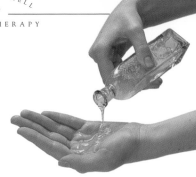

tea tree (*pp.24–5*) to a hot bath at the first sign of illness. Also use in steam inhalation.

INSOMNIA 🍃

Lavender (*pp.22–3*) and chamomile (*pp.42–3*), sandalwood (*pp.50–51*), rose (*pp.46–7*) and/or ylang ylang (*pp.40–41*). Use in a warm bath at bedtime, in massage, or in a vaporizer. Try 2 drops of lavender (*pp.22–3*) on a tissue tucked under your pillow.

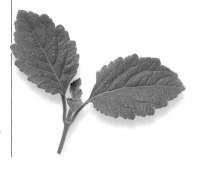

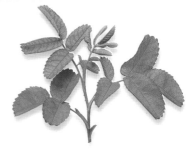

ME

Tea tree (pp.24–5) strengthens the immune system, rosemary (pp.26–7) has a tonic effect, geranium (pp.32–3) is an antidepressant. Massage is best where possible, but baths and vaporizers are also useful.

NAUSEA AND VOMITING

Relieve with lavender (pp.22–3), chamomile (pp.42–3), peppermint (pp.36–7), rose (pp.46–7), or sandalwood (pp.50–51) applied on a warm compress laid over the stomach. Gently massage over the stomach area. Use in a vaporizer.

NEURALGIA

Use lavender (pp.22–3), chamomile (pp.42–3), rosemary (pp.26–7), geranium (pp.32–3), clary sage (pp.28–9), or eucalyptus (pp.30–31) in the bath or most effectively on a hot compress applied to the affected area.

PERIOD PROBLEMS

• Heavy: geranium (pp.32–3), chamomile (pp.42–3), frankincense (pp.44–5), rose (pp.46–7).

• Irregular: clary sage (pp.28–9), chamomile (pp.42–3), lavender (pp.22–3), peppermint (pp.36–7), rose (pp.46–7).

• Scanty: lavender (pp.22–3), peppermint (pp.36–7), rose (pp.46–7).

• Painful: clary sage (pp.28–9), geranium (pp.32–3), lavender (pp.22–3), chamomile (pp.42–3), rose (pp.46–7). Use in a bath, in massage, and as a compress.

PMS

Clary sage (pp.28–9), lavender (pp.22–3), and chamomile (pp.42–3). Use rosemary (pp.26–7) and geranium (pp.32–3) for fluid retention and bloating. For irritability and depression choose rose (pp.46–7) and chamomile (pp.42–3). Use in massage, a bath, and a vaporizer.

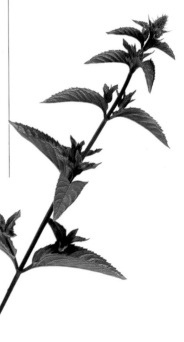

PSORIASIS

Sedative and antidepressant oils such as lavender (*pp.22–3*) and chamomile (*pp.42–3*) can help to reduce the stress that exacerbates the condition. Use in a bath, massage, and skin creams.

STRESS

Use any of the sedative oils to help you relax, e.g., lavender (*pp.22–3*), chamomile (*pp.42–3*), rose (*pp.46–7*), clary sage (*pp.28–9*) in a bath or in massage. For short periods of stress try rosemary (*pp.26–7*), geranium (*pp.32–3*), or peppermint (*pp.36–7*).

THRUSH

Baths, massage, and local applications of antifungal oils such as lavender (*pp.22–3*), tea tree (*pp.24–5*), myrrh, geranium (*pp.32–3*), and bergamot for vaginal thrush. Use a mouthwash made with myrrh for oral thrush.

VARICOSE VEINS

Cypress, lemon (*pp.34–5*), rosemary (*pp.26–7*), lavender (*pp.22–3*), or juniper used in a bath or compress. They can be mixed with a skin cream and rubbed gently over the area. If using massage, work gently below the affected area, never above. Vary your choice of oils.

Further reading

THE ILLUSTRATED ENCYCLOPEDIA OF ESSENTIAL OILS by *Julia Lawless* (Element)

AROMATHERAPY AN A–Z by *Patricia Davis* (CW Daniel)

PRACTICAL AROMATHERAPY by *Shirley Price* (Thorsons)

THE FRAGRANT PHARMACY by *Valerie Ann Worwood* (Bantam)

THE FRAGRANT MIND by *Valerie Ann Worwood* (Doubleday)

AROMATHERAPY BLENDS AND REMEDIES by *Franzesca Watson* (Thorsons)

PRINCIPLES OF AROMATHERAPY by *Cathy Hopkins* (Thorsons)

HEALTH ESSENTIALS: AROMATHERAPY by *Christine Wildwood* (Element)

Useful addresses

FOR INFORMATION

Aromatherapy Organizations Council
3 Latymer Close, Braybrooke
Market Harborough
Leicester LE16 8LN
Tel: 01858 434242

Aromatherapy Trade Council
PO Box 52, Market Harborough
Leicester LE16 8ZX
Tel: 01858 465731

American Alliance of Aromatherapy
PO Box 750428, Petaluma,
CA 94975–0428 USA
Tel: 1 707 778 6762
Fax: 1 707 769 0868

American Aromatherapy Association
PO Box 3679, South Pasadena
CA 91031 USA
Tel: 1 818 457 1742

National Association of Holistic Aromatherapy
PO Box 17622, Boulder
CO 80308–0622 USA
Tel: 1 303 258 3791

TO FIND A PRACTITIONER

International Federation of Aromatherapists
Stamford House
2–4 Chiswick High Road
London W4 1TH
Tel: 0181 742 2602
(Send an A5 s.a.e. and a cheque for £2 for a list of practitioners)